Trauma Healing Options for VA Hospitals

Help for Veterans to Own Their Healing and Their Future

Reverend Mike Wanner

Dedication

Trauma Healing Options for VA Hospitals

This book is dedicated to all those who have served to defend the United States of America and their families who have served also by missing them during their service and some forever. These valiant citizens have given freely in the pursuit of the noble goals specified in the Declaration of Independence and the Constitution of The United States and all the amendments thereto.

Special recognition is offered to those who have been injured or killed in the service of our country. The citizens now and future citizens of the United States of America will be forever in their debt. May all who have served be blessed in the now and the forever AND SO IT IS!

May All who Read this book be Blessed

Reverend Mike Wanner

Table of Contents

Introduction

We stand at a crossroads between the American Dream and American Reality. In the transition are the lives of many veterans who have served well and are entitled to the best that we have to offer.

What we have to offer veterans is the best that our society has endorsed through the professionals in various accrediting or oversight organizations. All this is appropriate according to the standards that we have set as operating criteria for the professionals.

What is not allowed for in our current system is the societal shifts of emotionality that have occurred. Neither the VA or traditional health care systems are equipped to deal with the emotional crisis that is still developing.

I believe that the addition of Spiritual Energy Therapies to the existing system can enhance effectiveness so that all veterans, citizens and practitioners can enjoy a new integrated system.

Chapter One

Veterans Desire to

Return to a Normal Life

After military service, many veterans crave a return to "normal" Life but it isn't easy for them to adapt. The good news is that the Veterans Administration provides tremendous resources to help the veterans along.

What is Normal?

Normal means different things to different people. The human condition is adaptable but adjusting to civilian life can be much more complicated than it sounds like it would be.

Peace of Mind

The Veterans Administration provides access to the top professionals in all categories so that clinical excellence is available for the asking. The culture of the military seems to make it difficult to ask and that can prove a huge hurdle for veterans to comprehend and cross.

Medical Care

It seems culturally Ok to Ask for Physical Support as in Medical Care. There seems to be justice when one has been physically hurt so that the military has an obligation to fix, support or treat the problem.

Acute Mental Issues

When a veteran has a mental crisis that is acute and debilitating, again accepting care is an obvious course of action. Treatment in Veterans Administration Hospitals or other treatment facilities can be arranged.

The Stigma of Disconnection

In every city, the news media talks about homeless veterans who are out in all kinds of weather. What is the issue with homeless veterans? There is a sort of disconnect or a series of disconnects that keeps these Veterans separate from the general population and many times, separate from other veterans.

One View

When talking to a fellow veteran at the Philadelphia VA Medical Center, I noticed that the gentlemen had obvious mental issues. At a poignant point in the conversation, I asked a distancing question about how "that" might be helped by a behavior consult for someone else in a hypothetical scenario.

My conversation partner was quick to point out the vulnerability that might exist for that person in not being able to find a job.

He felt that a diagnosis that would be needed to get support and care would actually be detrimental to the return to the normal world because the diagnosis would declare that the veteran might be a potential loose cannon who could pose a threat to workplace safety.

When I heard this, I balked in my head but remained quiet in my demeanor. The conversation ended when he was called for his appointment. I was saddened by the experience but glad that I understood a little more about his journey.

How My Journey Started

While my service was easy for the most part, there were scary times along the way. Back at the start, most new military members complain about basic training which went well for me. Technical school was a whole different story.

I was assigned to a student squadron which was notorious for being the sharpest looking squadron on the base. The reason it was sharp looking was because every man in it was afraid of what would happen if they were not. It was nicknamed the suicide squadron but the discipline was explained as "he fell down the stairs".

Our once comfortable fatigues held a crease pressed with a combination of Floor Polish and Starch. We walked funny because the legs were rigid like boards. Every spare minute was worked to be sharp and not get in trouble.

 Our soft sided work boots were turned in to rigid hard shells that could hold a spit shine. The pores in the leather were burnt shut with alcohol soaked cotton balls on the outside so the toes curled up and floor waxed on the inside so they could hold a shine and be rigid. It was hard to walk because the floor wax made the inside like a thorn bush.

Eventually they court marshalled the Squadron Commander and the First Sergeant and moved us to newly created school squadrons. We went from one extreme to the other.

I was then assigned permanent party to a base in West Texas where I did well and was selected for a special assignment that led to me cross training into maintenance control in Illinois. Later, I left Texas for Vietnam.

My Own Journey Back From Vietnam

My return to home was different than many as I did not have physical injuries that needed care at the VA. My return home was not smooth but like so many veterans, I self-medicated with alcohol and I could easily function. A cigarette addiction also helped to ease the mental pain that I would not acknowledge.

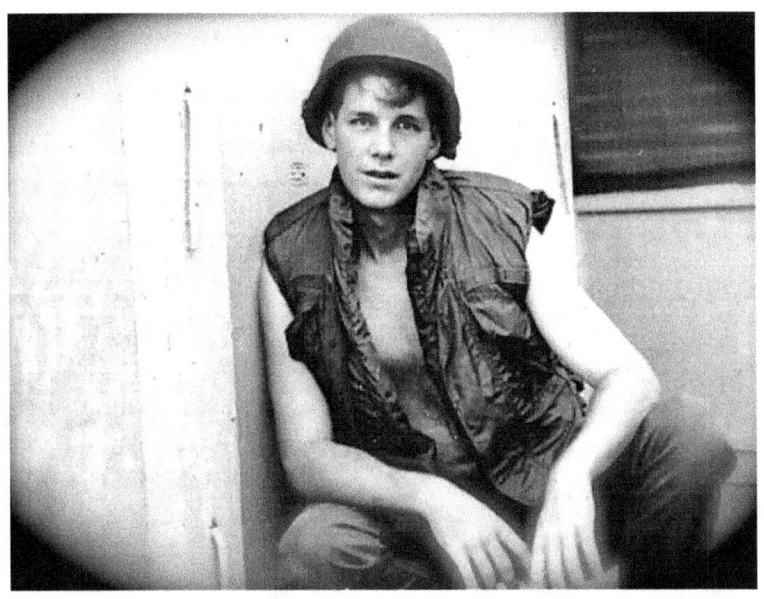

While my service was easy for the most part, I will always remember a certain close call to get to a bunker where I went into a suffocation-like anxiety that freaked out me and many others. The sweaty bodies huddled together against dirty dark sandbags in the stinging heat added a claustrophobic response to the anxiety.

Whenever I fly, I remember the transport flight back from Rest & Recuperation where our plane was hit taking off and the flight engineer in the C123 (an antique plane then which looked like 1/4 of a C130) came down and tied a big rope around his middle. He then opened the back of the plane by dropping the loading ramp in the rear to about 1/2 down. It seemed like control cables were everywhere hanging down and then he started counting cables that were still connected at both ends.

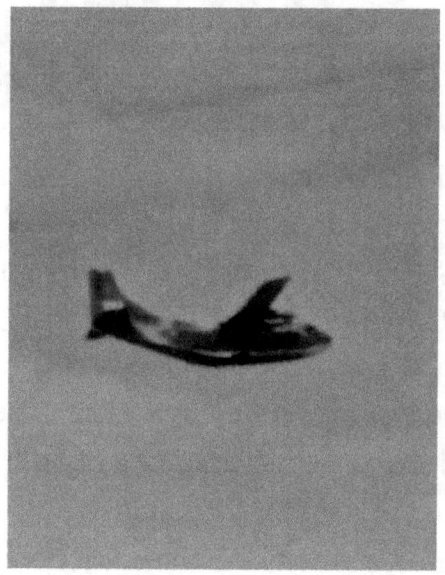

A stern look on his face broadened to a little smile as he looked around and said "I think we might do it". The flying time was short but the anticipation was palpable.

We all held our breath as we came in for an ever so long slow descent. Getting close to the ground, we suddenly fell like an elevator and we were all shocked by the impact of our landing. The ground has never been more welcome before or since.

I was the Precision Measuring Equipment Monitor for Nhatrang Air Base, Vietnam which was a workload control function of the Chief of Maintenance and my job was to insure that every piece of test equipment that calibrated anything was perfectly calibrated on a precise schedule. This proved very interesting and an unusual part of the job was hosting a field calibration team from the Cam Ranh Bay Precision Measuring Equipment Laboratory.

During their visit I needed to get them to Armed Forces Radio and TV Network station on top of Entre Island in the Bay of Nhatrang. I arranged for us to be on the supply landing craft.

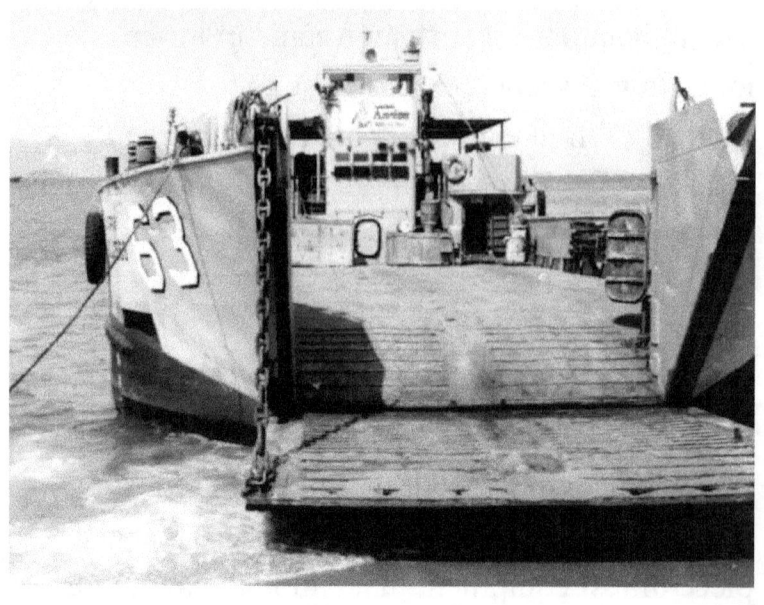

I did not arrange for the Typhoon which hit within hours of our arrival. I did not expect the orders from the island commander to help sandbag the roof. Two first aid injuries that day as my legs were scraped by jagged sections of the roof. Our planned one day visit was extended and proved a real rugged adventure since the island was merely a narrow steep mountain in the bay and everything was being blown and washed downhill.

Christmas in Vietnam was unexpectedly quiet. A way to cope for many military is to sing along with anybody who creates a song. One song we sang interferes briefly many times every Christmas. Whenever I hear Jingle Bells, my first reaction is the Vietnam words come up. We sang – Jingle Bells, Mortar Shells, VC in the grass, they can take this …..war and …………

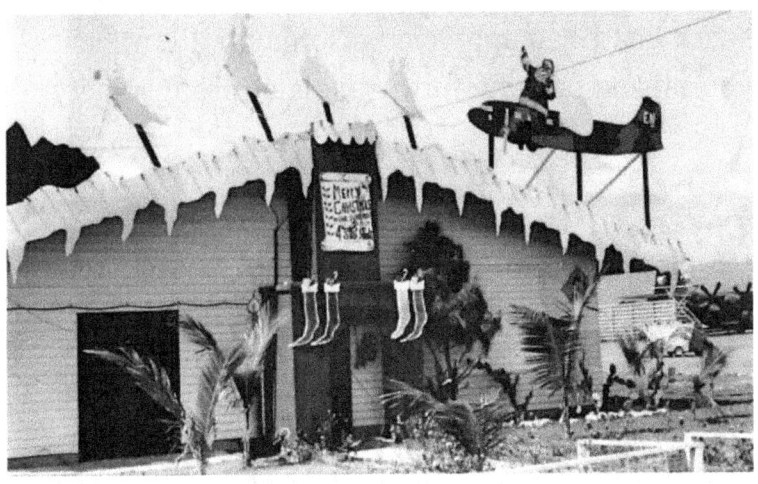

I Applied For VA Benefits

I applied for and was turned down for VA benefits. I accepted that and went about my life. Vietnam veterans were not warmly welcomed home so I did not feel the rejection was unusual.

Returning to Civilian Religion

The Military Chaplaincy Service had provided tremendous support for all of those at the bases where I was stationed. When I returned home, I was appalled to hear the gospel according to the checkbook that completely lacked the spiritual spark that I had appreciated so much. I left the church and became further isolated from society.

The Need to be of Service

I felt the loss of spiritual connectivity and felt most comfortable with those that were in pain. I was lead to a volunteer community ambulance program where I found purposeful activity that helped people. I still belong to that organization more than 45 years later.

Gaps in the volunteer service availability led me to start a professional Ambulance Company that kept me busy for twenty-five years. As Health Care became more complicated, I parted as I was being called into the world of spiritual energy.

Gift of God

In 1993, I was drawn to an alternative healing modality called Reiki which rekindled my spiritual motivation. I took a course offered at a center being run by a group of nuns who were doctors and nurses who ran medical programs of all kinds for the poor around the world.

The Medical Mission Sisters are fabulous examples of spiritual doers. I liked their style. Three years later, I joined the faculty at their wellness center and replaced my original Reiki Teacher. I went on to teach Reiki and other programs until they had to close twelve years later.

Back to the VA

In 2009, I was contacted by the VA and advised that I did qualify for VA Services after all. They scheduled my initial visit and then a specialty consult and I started getting some treatments.

Coming to Philadelphia VA was a wonderful experience and I felt like something that was poorly finished was suddenly OK again. I felt connected.

I went for a stress workshop and ironically everybody else did not show and I chatted with the counselor and a lot of feelings flooded my awareness. Things that I had not wanted to talk about for four decades were all of a sudden flowing and I felt great.

The feelings were so good that I started thinking that I might have some PTSD that had not cleared so I asked for an evaluation. The consult went well and I got to share a few episodes of my life which had been held in so long.

The counselor decided that these things were minimal and did not rise to the level of needing treatment. Of course, I had been working on them for forty years so that might have helped some.

Some Things that Helped Me

I honestly don't think that I would have regained my personal peace and connection with Creator if spiritual energy therapies like Reiki, Integrated Energy Therapy, Dowsing, Angel Healing, Channeling, Reiju, and Magnified Healing had not been found. My purpose in writing this is to share what has helped me.

I have read lately that the VA is getting creative in using alternative therapies to try and breakthrough the kind of disconnects that have been experienced by myself and others. I believe that Spiritual Energy Therapies can open many doors for veterans to reclaim a more peaceful level of normal at the earliest time possible.

What Can Help You/Others?

If you are or know a veteran who has felt disconnected, you are invited to share what the world needs to know. Especially welcome are comments about what safe topics you might come out to listen to or participate in. What is the non-physical wound that hurts?

Fear not for you are only alone if you choose to be.

I have shared what helped me. Please feel free to write me at mikewann@voicenet.com or leave comments on the veterans tab at http://AngelRaphaelSpeaks.com

I believe there are many veterans that are carrying heavy energy that has crimped their normal connection with God so much that they question their sanity.

I delight in working with folks who are ready to breakthrough on a spiritual basis and see that life has a lot of joy to offer us all because that is the gift we have been given.

*

Chapter Two
The Traditional Care Model

Traditionally we think of Body, Mind and Spirit as the categories of care and the providers of those Professional Services are Licensed and Credentialed persons.

Body Practitioners are Medical Doctors and Specialists. Mind Practitioners are Psychiatrists and Psychologists. Spiritual Practitioners are Ministers, Priests, Rabbis and other leaders according to the beliefs.

Each practitioner has their specialty and there is professional oversight by accrediting agencies or associations. i.e. The American Medical Association, the American Dental Association etc.

While the agencies above provide valuable controls over their membership that protects the interests of us all, it is difficult to provide guidelines for populations as diverse as there are.

It is my hope, that the traditional model can be enhanced by the VA experience. Lessons learned helping to bridge un-seeable gaps that are showing up for veterans can also help in the general ability to help all cope with the intensity of current times.

Chapter Three
The Human Factor

Separate from the clinical perspectives shared by each specialty, the client needs to advocate for their own sense of values. Herein lies the potential for a problem as the self-confidence of many is lacking and there is a possibility that the patient/client may not be assertive enough to have their feelings understood.

Safety is a significant issue for veterans and that is a quite natural situation in that there is essentially conflict in that which one has been trained to believe at different points in their life. When one was in school, there was training about being well behaved and adhering to certain community codes of conduct.

When one grew up and entered the service, the expectations of them were directed and the means to achieve those goals were specific. Once entering an environment that lacked the safety of one's upbringing with rules that did not match their peace and tranquility, times could easily be called stressful.

Later upon discharge, the same person is expected to change again to a new situation that has rules that may be the same as the original rules but are really quite different in that the person is no longer the same person that lived in those rules previously.

Being in an environment where one can be heard, accepted and understood even casually is very comforting. For me, it was many years before I heard the words welcome home and felt that my service in Vietnam was appreciated.

Chapter Four
The Family Doctor

In a bygone era, family doctors could spend a lot more time with their patients and understand the total person. Survival for doctors now requires them to comply with the industry practices.

Unfortunately we assign to those delightful servants of humanity the many things that are better handled by ourselves and others. Their time with us is very precious and they have to work within expected protocols and criteria.

In just the last fifty years family doctors have been bombarded with responsibility. They are usually expected to create marvelous results at minimal costs.

Life has accelerated in the last fifty years and many of the natural things that have helped doctors in the past are not resources now.

Quality of life issues alone have changed the way we live. Drug addiction, genetically modified foods, violence in the homes and war ramifications have created problems that are difficult if not impossible for doctors to treat.

Chapter Five
The Emotional Self

There is no longer time for us to continue to avoid the emotional realties of our times. As a population, emotionality is out of control and that is clearly shown by the rapid spread of divorce and drug abuse.

That which has been relied on for ages to mark the path for us to walk is now clouded by the emotions that are raging with the populations of the world.

Taking Responsibility

In your personal life, the strongest things that you can do is get a grip on your life by taking responsibility for everything in it and choosing how it should be.

Chapter Six

A New Perspective Is Needed

Physical Care

Physical Care is the domain of the Medical Doctor. The general practitioner that we all see is for most of us the gatekeeper for our care. We routinely surrender responsibility for our care to him or her.

While they take this trust seriously, over time there has been a cultural dynamic where we surrender too much responsibility to the good doctors and don't take any responsibility ourselves. This is bad on so many levels.

Consider that Doctors only have about 25% of the authority that we do. They have a license to practice medicine and that pertains to only about a quarter of the total care we need. The doctors have the physical area to practice medicine. But we are physical and emotional and mental and spiritual beings.

Unfairly, we have frequently expected doctors to fix everything. They do not have the authority to practice outside their level of licensure.

The emotional and mental and spiritual elements of us remain our responsibility to integrate and unfortunately many of us do not understand that and we go and sue a Doctor for our malpractice of being us.

Emotional Care

The term emotional care means different things to different people and there are frequently supporters who are really enablers which support the characteristics of the one being supported in a way that is not healthy.

Just being around and listening to someone is not always helpful to healing and growth. If one encounters a drug addict who needs a fix and wants to help, giving them money for drugs is not the answer. Conversely this type of support is detrimental.

Emotional support is about balance and perspective. It is about weighing all the issues and making balanced thoughtful decisions that are congruent with one's personal values.

Mental Care

The mind is a simple and complicated asset that can bring us understanding and balance. The mind can also delude us in to thinking that things are different than they really are and cause us to respond according to what we think there is instead of what there is in reality.

Positivity is essential to keep one focused and upbeat so that the normal issues of life are dealt with in a balanced way.

Spiritual Care

The disconnect for many people between the physical realm and the spiritual world can be vast. Many do not realize that the absence of a spiritual connection means that the total support system is not optimized.

God can seem elusive to many people but in reality, God is the constant and we are the ones that may drift away from the blessings that are available to all at all times. When we take the initiative and invite God, the reconnection is immediate and complete.

Chapter Seven

Four Parts To Healing

It has become clear to me that we are missing some signals and may be headed in the wrong direction. I would be remiss if I did not offer my observations about common sense things that the citizens of the world can do to help improve the postures for their success, survival and sustenance.

We each Need Four Support Systems

Tables supported by four legs are usually pretty stable. We are each like a table in that we need support to keep us on an even level.

We each need support for the total Body, Mind and Spirit of our experience and in earlier easier times, those three kinds of support were enough to keep us going. In todays' complex circumstances, We need to add an emotional support to the structure.

Chapter Eight

Life Isn't Easy

A prevalent element of modern culture shows victimization as acceptable and usable to justify limited performance, the need for others to pay attention to us and other socially unacceptable behavior. Those that are victimized by others use that as a defense to justify the victimization of others.

We each have the capacity to rise out of our own ashes like a Phoenix, to create for ourselves a new beginning. Regardless of most of what we have endured before now, we can transform ourselves and our lives. Perhaps, the true purpose of suffering is to learn that from our pain we can rise, expand, grow, achieve and thrive.

Subtle Options

Subtle energy modalities have spoken to me as the best alternatives for dealing with the human condition so that we can stay out of crisis.

I am writing as if a mandate was issued that I do this. The words Quantum Quatro had been coming to me for some time and an early push start to a busy day demanded that paper be filled with my thoughts.

A heavy daily schedule could be smoothed if we each take a little time to support each leg of our powerful subtle system.

Chapter Nine

Welcome to Quantum Quatro! Subtle Energy System Support

While the title is a bit much, the concept is very simple. If we want to heal, we need to deal with all four segmented human needs as they interrelate within a healthy person.

This chapter is about the Four Support Systems that we need to keep balanced in our lives. The systems are:

............Physical Support

.........Emotional Support

.............Mental Support

............Spiritual Support

Each of these areas is significant because they all interact on an ongoing basis and if one loses lift then the unified you is tweaked and that is not healthy. On the next three pages, I will offer an example of a method below for each area that needs to be supported. Other Methods may be just as effective.

Physical Support System

A system called Reiki while a gift from the Divine for our total existence has a most powerful impact on things related to the physical body and the healing thereof. Reiki can be a big part of all healing and if you only have Reiki in your tool bag, you have a lot. An advanced Reiki system called Karuna Reiki focuses on compassion and when you develop it for others, the compassion for yourself is surprisingly beneficial.

Reiki can be used in person or sent at a distance to the one needing it.

Emotional Support Systems

An energy modality called Integrated Energy Therapy has changed my life. It allows one to invoke angelic energy for the release of stuffed emotions and cellular memory. The process has the practitioner establish an angelic heartlink with angel energy and then work on nine cellular memory areas of a person in a process of energizing and integrating the energies there.

Integrated Energy Therapy can be used in person or sent at a distance to the one needing it.

Mental Support System

Our minds can be our strongest ally or our weakest link. When we allow our minds to just run, there seems to be a great cloud of possibilities on a scale from good to evil. When we take charge of our minds and direct them to a focus then we can move toward that goal. Sorting through the many questions can be daunting. The best resource that I have found so far is an ancient system called Dowsing that allows me to quickly run through possibilities and objectively help clients find goals that resonate with a progressive path out of an apparent state of overwhelming emotional paralysis.

Dowsing can be done in person or at a distance.

Spiritual Support Systems

Prayer is Powerful and its' ability is increased with frequency. The frequency can be in that the person saying the prayer says more or it can be that the assistance of a person of prayer, a minister, a prayer circle, a prayer therapist or an on-line distant healing group can add to the efforts of the prayer. One great resource for prayer support is the webpage www.Create-A-Prayer.com.

Prayer can be practiced in person or at a distance.

Chapter Ten

The Importance of the VA Hospital System

The VA Hospital is a National Resource not only for caring for veterans but in the development and integration on techniques, protocols and equipment that other hospitals cannot justify in the civilian health care marketplace.

Addiction is plaguing many veterans but it is also plaguing many civilians and when a breakthrough is attained in the VA Medical Centers, we all benefit in many ways.

Stories about the VA reaching out for alternative and complementary methods are encouraging because as success is found, more efforts will be initiated.

The Beauty of many of the modalities that I would like to suggest is that they can be implemented with little infrastructure and minimal personnel. The existent chaplain system may be incentivized to expand in to some of the roles suggested.

I hope the veterans get the opportunities to grow from the ability to choose some of these options.

Chapter Eleven
The Emotional Puzzle

As one who had an early childhood parental loss, I had long suppressed my struggle to understand why things were the way they were. The military added structure to my life which was well received initially.

I never really understood the complete impact of my loss until I had a soul retrieval performed by a shaman that I trusted. She made it clear to me that the automatic mantra that paralyzed me in certain situations was really just a habit that I could control at will.

The lesson learned in the soul retrieval allowed me to form a perspective of the situation that I could later implement in to my energy treatments for clients.

A tremendously effective tool in the field was found when I integrated energy pullout techniques of Integrated Energy Therapy with identification of the age when an issue started for someone. It was so elementary to just clearly identify the issue and the emotion that was troublesome to the client and then use Dowsing to determine an age when the trouble started.

I called the result - the Age Of Cause and am still amazed when I ask someone what happened at the age that I dowsed. The answer is typically – nothing.

Time allows the seed of the question to percolate and sometime later, the person will contact me and say what happened then. Equipped with the personal energy clues, I can then move forward quite quickly to help melt the energy blockages that are an issue.

The release of an energy blockage can really empower somebody.

Everybody Is Different

Hearing my story does not give you answers to the problems in your life or the lives of your friends or clients. Everybody has a different history and that leads to them having different challenges or opportunities.

Many answers came for me when I tapped in to the spiritual side of myself. Please notice that I said spiritual and not religious as I want to make a clear distinction between the two.

Religious practice is rooted in the doctrine of the many different religions that individuals follow. Spirituality is about a one on one connection between you and the Divine – A Direct Line to God.

Listening is the big tool for learning. Many will tell you that you have been born with two ears and one mouth and you should follow that by listening twice as much as you speak. Excellent advice still.

Everybody Chooses

When you are listening to others, you have the opportunity to learn about how they process and from them you can learn more about how you do it. When you see where they have an opportunity to create an optional outcome, you can also see that you have options in your life.

Have you made the right choices in your life? Would you go back if you could and change some things.

The truth is that the minute that you read this is the first minute of the rest of your life and you can make new choices that will take you to a new place in your future.

This may sound good but seem impossible to do. It is understandable if a piece of you will be whispering that it is impossible for you to have that much power. Fear not for you have great power available when you claim it.

Chapter Twelve
Empowerment

Empowerment is a process by which many veterans can find their way back to their power. The way to accomplish empowerment is as broad as the veterans who might want to claim it.

My goal here is not to answer all the questions about how everybody can be saved from everything. Instead, I wish to add some resources to the systemic excellence that already exists.

Some of the veterans that are in the disconnected category can very well be the recruiters that are needed to go out and help those that are even more disconnected. The goal then is to create an opportunity for options to be heard that can be more inclusive than what has been already tried.

Thoughts are things and can create new possibilities for service to many who have been un-served so far.

Chapter Thirteen
Reintegration

The Invitations Have Been Sent

The welcome mat is out and the word has gone out. Is the invitation correct?

Will the invited be greeted in a way that can be accepted by them? Perhaps. Who knows?

It may be that we need a motivational connection that will help those that are still unconnected to find their way. Perhaps there is the need for a draw. And what would that be?

New Ideas Aplenty

I will include a list of my ideas but that is only a beginning. The creativity of many is needed here now so that we can revitalize an effort to learn from the past and prepare for the future in a new way that benefits all.

It is likely that each segment of the military could have career field pertinent outreaches that can provide for the grounding of new groups of veterans. The facilities already exist which can host many small groups that can be the first step in the saving of the quality of many lives.

Let the available facilitators and organizers be the ones to show how the next steps should go.
This can be initiated on a very progressive basis when a beginning point can be found.

Chapter Fourteen
Starting Ideas

Story Time

When you talk to veterans long enough, stories come out that help to heal and honor the members of the Army, Air Force, Navy, Marines, Coast Guard and National Guard. Story time can be organized as a general session or specific as to a branch of the service.

Spouse Story Time

Behind many veterans are spouses who have served their own personal missions as supporters of the veteran and their families. Support for aging veterans may have spouses looking for ideas from other spouses who have been attached to a veteran.

Writing Class

Writing offers a powerful way to transfer feelings to paper which can be very therapeutic. The structure of a class can also provide a community connection that many may need to reconnect.

Once written, reading their work can further bond them to their classmates and help them go deeper into themselves so they can find more opportunities to shine.

Spiritual Poetry Reading

Many poems have been written of a spiritual nature. Having a session where individuals can share their favorite stories can be very helpful to focus on positive possibilities.

Angel Stories

Talking about Angels has a way of grabbing the interest of many individuals and then they can begin to think about higher vibration topics that can serve them well on the journey to healing.

Perhaps there can be both reading and writing segments to the sessions.

Hospital Healing Stories

Angel in the Laundry

I do Pastoral Visitations at a dynamic Philadelphia hospital which is next to the elevated tracks in a mature area of the city that hosts tremendous diversity.

When I came in to a hospital room this day, I recognized a frequent flyer and she was happy to see me. I asked why she was there and was told that she had a heart attack two days before. She also said she was having a good day today. I asked why? She told me the story.

Months earlier, she was in the same hospital and someone brought her a beautiful Angel pin. It meant a lot to her because it was given at a low point in her situation. In the excitement of being discharged, she grabbed up her belongings and went home. When she looked for the Angel, it could not be found.

That day before my visit, she had some bleeding and the nurses cleaned her up. When she was clean, a little nurse went out to the laundry cart and grabbed a fresh gown and brought it to her.

After the nurse helped her put it on, she smoothed out the garment and there was her Angel Pin. The questions abound about how this could be. Only one answer makes sense.

It is that when God sends a message, the rules of time and space don't matter. Great things happen at Great Hospitals!

> Rev. Mike Wanner
> Circle of Miracles Minister
> 4/26/07

The Man Shaking From Head to Toe

I went to do a pastoral visit on this day and as I entered the room I saw a man who was shaking from head to toe. I introduced myself and asked if there was something that he wanted to Pray About (Pause), Talk About (Pause) or Complain about.

He laughed a shallow laugh but it was enough. He told me a story of disconnection from God because of his human experience with the church and why he could not go back. I explained to him that Philadelphia was a big city and if he didn't like that priest, he could go to another church or denomination until he found one suitable.

Making no headway I told him about an exercise that I share called the Hand Up Handout. We did the exercise and he stopped shaking.

After lunch, I was walking past the room and I noticed that his hand was up in the air and I went in to check. I reminded him that once he reconnected with God, he could put his hand down. His reply was NOT YET!

Here is the Hand Up Handout

When things seem bad, it is very natural to feel down in the dumps and isolated and cutoff. There is both a physical and psychological dynamic to this isolation and the trauma that it supports.

I have found that the simple act of reaching the left, or receiving hand, up to God during prayer seems to make an awesome difference in the experience of all people and especially those that are depressed. The action taken seems to break them free of patterns of limited thinking and enables them to reconnect to the God that loves them so much.

Prayer by itself to many seems hollow because there is an expectation that nothing will happen but when they reach out and up there is a shift, an expectancy that things will be different. That expectancy breaks through some sort of mental disconnect obstruction mechanism and allows the mental obstacles to dissipate.

I find the Hand Up most effective when used with a customized prayer. The connection occurs within a second and the hand can be relaxed.

I invite you to reach out for breakthroughs in your life by connecting with the strongest power that there is – your creator.

I invite you to share this with those that need to be lifted up. Your caring and this technique may make the first shift that they have had in a long time .

May all who read this be blessed,
AND SO IT IS.

Rev. Mike

StressReleaseCoach.com
215-342-1270
E-mail: mikewann@voicenet.com

Chapter Fifteen
Energy Medicine

An emerging field of study called energy medicine is may have some roots in the spiritual Energy modalities that have been so successful for many years.

I would encourage further development of a discussion on energy medicine throughout the VA Medical community.

The beauty of energy medicine is that much of it can be done by the patients themselves or their families or bodywork practitioners.

A number of the techniques can be investigated to provide personal experiences for veterans that can help them know that they can achieve a new normal that is aligned with them Being at peace.

I will add some of these systems as separate chapters that the VA can consider individually.

There is much more to be researched. I share that which I know and can talk about.

Chapter Sixteen
Reiki

A wonderful healing modality has circled the world. It is called Reiki and is traced back to Mikao Usui of Japan. This great man has done a lot for Japanese relations with the world. I am one who appreciates him tremendously and there are many that practice his teachings. I would hope that all the world could learn of this gift. I would like to think that the Japanese people understand how great a person he was. I am grateful to his homeland for contributing to his personhood. May all the Japanese learn of his great teachings and allow the method to help them.

What does Reiki Mean

REI means "Universal" or "Spiritually Guided"
KI means "Life Force" or "Energy
Pronounced as "Ray-Key"

Reiki is Natural Energy that is:

1. A healing method that is non-invasive

2. An agent for personal expansion and change
3. A spiritual path of service
4. A compliment to all other accepted healing methods.

Reiki is not:

A substitute for Medical care.
A substitute for Emotional Care and/or Support
A substitute for Psychological/Psychiatric Care.
A substitute for Spiritual Care.
A massage technique
A religion or cult.

Reiki is applied by:
Laying hands on or close to a person.
Transmission from a distance.

Reiki can:
Revitalize and energize.
Relieve stress and body tension.
Accelerate healing
Calm the mind.
Stimulate spiritual awareness
Aid in balancing emotions.
Be an agent of change.
Help to dissipate energy blockages.
Be a spiritual path.

Reiki is the channeling of the life force that flows through all living things. It is a natural healing technique that uses laying-on of hands and other energy transference methods to transfer or channel this energy. The first part of the word "Rei" means "Universal" or "Spiritually guided" and "Ki" means life force or energy.

It is believed that Reiki originated thousands of years ago but it's use for physical healing was lost or held secret for most of the last twenty centuries

One great thing about Reiki is it's simplicity. Anybody can do it, even me, even you and yes, even children. There are no special skills required. As long as you can form the intention to channel the energy, you can do Reiki.

I once had the privilege to start a Reiki program at Siloam which was dedicated to Wellness through spirituality in the HIV/Aids community. One Kids Reiki class there finished with four little children doing Reiki on their infected mother. The picture of mom's relaxation and pride was priceless.

Chapter Seventeen
Integrated Energy Therapy®

Integrated Energy Therapy is the most powerful energy modality that I have found to focus on clearing stuffed emotions and cellular memory. The system uses a powerful angelic heart connection called a Heartlink to establish a channel for the energy work to be accomplished.

You can find practitioners throughout the country and the world and right in your community. If you need help finding a practitioner, then you could go to the www.LearnIET.com site and look for instructors.

While it is a powerful modality to receive as a client of a practitioner, there is great healing ability for oneself when you choose to learn how to be a practitioner. There are three levels for practitioners - Basic, Intermediate and Advanced. There is also a Master Instructor level.

Chapter Eighteen
Magnified Healing

Magnified Healing® is a system that has a unique approach to healing in that the goal is to invite a constant flow of energy from the heart to source. The System claims the intervention and inspiration of Quan Yin , the goddess of mercy and compassion and the patron of women, for the expansion of the energy for the spiritual advancement of humanity and the earth.

My personal experience of Magnified Healing is that it is a devotional effort working in and through Quan Yin to facilitate healing throughout the people of the world and the world itself.

I was and still am fascinated by the sensations experienced when a participant is asking for a rewiring and reconnection of the nervous system.

Chapter Nineteen
Energy Messages for the Sick

The Situation May Be Overwhelming

The chaos of any moment may seem unfathomable. You may feel helpless but it is important to know that times like these are the times when the arms of God are available for you to fall into at will.

You Always Have Power Available To You!

Even when it seems hopeless, there is always something that we can do to help ourselves or those we love. Our thoughts have the ability to attract, create and activate great power.

Listen To People
Who Uplift your Spirit

Many people will come in to your life and each can have significant impact. It is up to you to determine who your friends will be and how much of their influence you will allow. It is important that you continue to think for yourself and align with the forces of goodness, wellness and harmony. Your personal peace helps you to be able to help others.

Find Out Where The One You
Want to Help is Emotionally

When I work with people, I want to know what they are feeling so that I can determine how to help them best. Realizing the power of emotions allows us to focus on integrating everything.

I test to prioritize the time that I have to spend with folks. I just ask them to give me a number (Tens

Scale 1-10) that measures their intention about a specific emotion and that tells me a lot.

Emotional Help for Healing

It is easy to get lost in traditional care regimens but the science is so powerful and necessary. Beside the clinical variables is a human being having a sickness experience that is totally new to them and confusing.

The emotionality alone can be problematic and can impede the natural process of healing. Besides the best in traditional care, emotional help for healing can be stress reduction, stress release, relaxation, spiritual support and energy healing modalities.

We Are Where We Are

The emotionality of illness is akin to the lost feeling that one can have when they get lost in a strange city. Personal peace finding is possible when you avoid the blaming, fault finding and anger by just accepting that you are where you are.

What Do We Do Next?

We can go it alone and continue to be lost or we can accept the situation and embrace the supernatural possibilities available to us. I recommend the latter.

The Affected and the Afflicted

If you are afflicted of affected, great power is available to you as long as you can form the intention to help every situation that involves you or anyone else. We are never really alone even when we feel that we are. God, our Creator, created us in love and loves us still.

In the depth of any darkness is huge potential to understand and align with the potential for good, health, wholeness and wellness. Your pain is an alarm system that tells you that something is wrong and that can be Physical, Emotional, Mental or Spiritual.

Allowing Love In

Many people have a huge problem with allowing love to come to them. The circumstances of their lives may make things less than clear and confuse actions as threats even when they were initiated with love.

Misunderstandings and personal defensiveness are breeding fields for illness that can be used by the dark forces of the universe to take people further from the Divine source of personal power. A spiral of darkness can enter the lives of the overwhelmed.

When illness strikes and we are forced to stop the whirlwind of modern day existence, it is a great time to reevaluate. If you are flat on your back, invite the power of God to help you.

The Geographical Disconnect

There seems to exist a geographical disconnect between humanity and God at times (A non-physical but perceivable mental disconnect between the physical world and the nonphysical). People get the idea that they are here on earth and God is in Heaven and we are not connected. Truth is lacking in that thinking.

Asking God for a Blessing

Many people pray for things and are not thrilled with the results. I invite you to consider praying to be a new improved you who might naturally attract good. That prayer is contingent upon you taking good actions and God supporting that action.

Praying For Others

Putting others first provides a natural reordering of your priorities and blesses many. You may find this helps you get over any resistance to asking for help. It also helps to keep the asker in a power place of prayer where you are in the Creator Light and dark forces do not wish to go there.

The Power of Prayer

I so believe in prayer that I have a whole web site dedicated to it. Consider visiting and learning how to structure your prayers so that they are personally optimized. Visit http://www.Create-A-Prayer.com.

You Can Work With God

I hope by now I have raised your awareness a little about what can be and now for the shocker. YOU CAN TAP IN TO THE AWESOME POWER OF

GOD. YES all are worthy if they just intend that they want to be a channel of GOD. We are all prewired with all that we need to do the job.

I have written extensively about the methods at our disposal but even without all that, we can invite and ground healing for ones we care about and ourselves.

The Still Small Voice
Speaks the Truth

The guidance within is extremely precise when we surrender all doubt and just ask to be shown. There is nothing that you can't do through God who strengthens you.

The Guidance Of An almighty God

So many people doubt their guidance because they do not feel the worthiness to do the bidding of the Divine. You are worthy because you were born worthy. You were born the cherished child of an awesome God. You are loved beyond measure and there is no expiration date or conditions upon which you will be separated from God at God's initiative.

The Power of Healing Systems

I cannot overemphasize the healing potential of the non-physical systems. While I do not for one minute minimize the power of traditional Health Care, I have to tell you that many churches of the world and the practitioners of spiritual healing have the ability to help you traverse the normal clinical borders that professional licensing boards establish and assist flawless integration that only an unlimited God could allow.

Living Your Life

If you drift toward God, your life will be in the flow of all that's good. I have a resources page that could give you many ideas. It is at the end of this book.

Will You Begin to Heal Yourself and the Sick

I sincerely hope that you will. As you do the work of God, you will know that it is making a difference. As your light shines bright in God's work, know that you will be a bigger target for temptation. Have no fear for you can prevail.

The Healing You Are Called to do

Do not wait for others to tell you how you can help. Ask in prayer and meditation for the guidance you seek and a knowing will come into your thoughts.

From your thoughts, guidance, experiences, questions, anxieties, decisions and ponderings will come a step that may not seem like guidance but will be just enough for you to take the next step on your path. Have no concerns about where you are going as long as you know in your heart that you are on the right path.

It is my prayer that your attraction to this section allows you to know at a deep level that you are called in service to help one or many whom your heart has recognized.

What is Possible?

You can do all things through God who strengthens you. Allow yourself to prepare now.

Reclaiming Your Power and Health

The answer is you. I have touched on some possibilities and have websites for you to read from and other resources on the following pages. You, like me, have been drawn in to the possibilities for us to help. The path might not be easy or clear but the Souls we have been given are calling us to fulfill our purpose of lovingly and completely nurturing the ones that we have been born to help. May all who read these words be blessed, uplifted and nurtured AND SO IT IS!

Chapter 20
Programs for The VA to Consider

The list of programs that follows is non-traditional and controversial and definitely not offered as a replacement for traditional care. The programs have a different base and may be effective for those individuals who are ready to approach their situation in a comprehensive way.

It is my hope that these programs will be effective in one or more ways;

> As a way to relaxation and reality.
> As a way to Spiritual Healing.
> As a way to open to Homeostasis.
> As a complement to the total VA system.

The major effect of Reiki and other spiritual Healing Modalities is to stimulate relaxation which can allow veterans to enter the desired state of being known as Homeostasis where healing opportunities are maximized in the relaxed adult.

Traditional Usui Reiki Classes

The VA could host or provide access to trainings for Veterans. Arrangements would be needed with a Reiki Master to facilitate that.

Traditional Usui Reiki Shares

The VA Could host or provide access for practitioners to do client sessions or shares for Veterans.

Crisis Reiki

Crisis Reiki is an adaptation of traditional Reiki for people who lack the time or the money to study traditional Reiki. I put up a whole website that discusses this practice and anyone can read about it at http://www.CrisisReiki.com

Baby Reiki

Baby Reiki is an adaptation of Crisis Reiki that invites women to prepare for childbirth by nurturing themselves and their fetuses with Reiki prior to and after birth.

Baby Reiki could be a wonderful gift from the VA to all service personnel when the wives are separated from the husband during pregnancy.

Reiju for You

Reiju for You – The attunement processes used to create Reiki practitioners can also be used as an empowerment process. Gendai Reiki has it as a part of the master curriculum but other lineages also have references for Healing attunements.

Breaking Mental Blocks

How many times have you heard someone say that they have a mental block about something. When thought forms attach to a persons' thinking, it can be difficult for those patterns to dissipate.

When the reality that thoughts are things is taken seriously, energy practitioners can help some people to move through mental blocks. This like all areas of energy work are not for everybody but they can be helpful to those that feel they are ready, willing and able to create newness in their life.

Breaking Mental Blocks can be as effective as shedding emotional baggage. Reiki and IET both offer help in this regard.

Clearing Cellular Memory

Cellular memory can be from this lifetime or past lifetimes and issues can be from either or a combination of both.

Stuffed Emotion Clearing

Veterans, probably more than any other group, can feel stuffed emotions that may cause them problems. Road rage is a civilian version of stuffed emotions. One can imagine what could happen to a veteran that has stuffed emotions and then has to deal with a citizen who is in road rage.

The times we live in are very intense and do not make it any easier for veterans.

Emotional Clearing Groups

Emotional clearing can be supported by group energy.

Angel Messages

For some the concept of Angels may be difficult to believe, others may find new levels of understanding. The author has channeled hundreds of messages from Angel Raphael and has free messages available on Facebook, and on http://www.AngelRaphaelSpeaks.com and on http://www.spiritualcomfortcare.com/angel-raphael-speaks/

Veterans & Veterans of the Streets

Inner city youth can have struggles of their own and it might be possible to introduce them to the VA in a way that is helpful to the vets, the kids, the VA and the cities. The stories of unconnected-ness may be very helpful to kindred spirits that are trying to survive in their respective challenges. Strategizing between the two groups could change lives.

Thought Surrender Workshops

Ideas about how to release thoughts and transfer energy could be held.

Listening workshops

The importance of being heard where Veterans could buddy up and talk.

Depression Lifting

Veterans could be introduced to the power of focused belief and or work with an Integrated Energy Therapist.

It Isn't That Simple

An ongoing workshop could be developed to explain the steps needed to attain progress in any part of the system.

Group Energy Focusing

Veterans could take turns sitting in a circle of friends and having the outer circle beam them with energy, prayer or good intentions.

Scientific Prayer Assembly

A scientific prayer assembly workshop could be developed around the principles available on my http://www.Create-A-Prayer-com website.

While the process is easily Do It Yourself, a group approach allows an acceptability that empowers.

Prayer Partnerships

Prayer partners could be encouraged where people take on the responsibility for praying for each other. Veterans could have more than one partner.

Chaplains may do the pairing or a simple list of people who want to participate or both.

Group Angel Channeling

Group channeling can be very helpful to participants. Everyone may not get the opportunity to ask but the energy of the gathering can create a community harmonic balance that is very soothing to all attendees. Even those who merely observe can have perspective shifting.

Chapter Twenty-One

Bible References For Healing

An Old Path to New Healing

This section is about connecting to the energy, light and healing you need when you seek wholeness. The acquisition of wholeness will be focused on and then referenced to a biblical reference of the process to attain it. We will see that the path to healing has been there for a long time but for many it is a trail that has not been found .

The Need to Let Go of Judgment

Jesus Christ clearly specified that we need freedom from the Judgment.

Matthew 7:1 "Judge not that ye be not judged"

Matthew 7:2 " For with what judgment ye judge, ye shall be judged: and with what measure ye mete, it shall be measured to you again. "

Letting Go of Excuses

Healing requires the letting go of excuses. We need to focus our attention on our own business. Our business of inviting healing in to our lives and the lives of those that we love.

Why should we look at that splinter in another's eye and ignore the one in ours? We should not. It is not productive.

Matthew 7:3 "And why beholdest thou the mote that is in thy brother's eye but considerest not the beam that is in thy own eye?"

Are you ready to focus on reality?

The Need for Communication with the Divine

All the goodness in life is available to those that ask the right source. What is it that you want? Are you willing to ask for it?

Luke 11:9 "And I say unto you, Ask, and it shall be given you; seek, and ye shall find; knock, and it shall be opened unto you."

Luke 11:10 "For every one that asketh receiveth; and he that seeketh findeth; and to him that knocketh it shall be opened."

The Power of Belief

After you have asked for what you want, you still have more to do, you need to maintain the belief that what you have asked for will manifest and then you have to hold that belief until it happens.

Matthew 9:20 "And, behold, a woman, which was diseased with an issue of blood twelve years, came behind him, and touched the hem of his garment:"

Matthew 9:21 "For she said within herself; If I may touch his garment, I shall be whole.

Matthew 9:22 "But Jesus turned him about and when he saw her, he said, Daughter, be of good comfort; Thy faith hath made thee whole. And the woman was made whole from that hour."

{Above also in Mark 5:25, 26, 27, 28 }

{Above also in Luke 8:43, 44, 45, 46, 47, 48}

*

Matthew 9:27 "And when Jesus departed thence, two blind men followed him, crying, and saying, Thou son of David, have mercy on us."

Matthew 9:28 "And when he was come into the house, the blind men came to him: and Jesus saith unto them, Believe ye that I am able to do this? They said unto him, Yea, Lord."

Matthew 9:29 "Then touched he their eyes, saying, According to your faith be it unto you."

The Power of Touch

Mark 1:40 "And there came a leper to him, beseeching him, and kneeling down to him, and saying unto him, If thou wilt, thou canst make me clean."

Mark 1:41 "And Jesus, moved with compassion, put forth his hand, and touched him, and saith unto him, I will: be thou clean."

{Above also in Matthew 8:2, 3}

{Above also in Luke 5:12, 13}

*

Matthew 8:14 "And when Jesus was come into Peter's house, he saw his wife's mother laid, and sick of a fever."

Matthew 8:15 "And he touched her hand, and the fever left her: and she arose, and ministered unto them."

Matthew 8:16 "When the even was come, they brought unto him many that were possessed with the devils: and he cast out the spirits with his word, and healed all that were sick:

Matthew 8:17 "That it might be fulfilled which was spoken by E-sa'-ias the prophet, saying. HIMSELF TOOK OUR INFIRMITIES, AND BARE OUR SICKNESSES."

{Above also in Mark 1:30, 31}

{Above also in Luke 4:38, 39}

*

Mark 6:56 "And whithersoever he entered, into villages, or cities, or country, they laid the sick in the streets, and besought him that they might touch if it were but the border of his garment: and as many as touched him were made whole."

{Above also in Matthew 14:36}

*

Mark 7:32 "And they bring unto him one that was deaf, and had an impediment in his speech: and they beseech him to put his hand upon him."

Mark 7:33 "And he took him aside from the multitude, and put his fingers into his ears, and he spit, and touched his tongue;"

Mark 7:34 "And looking up to heaven, he sighed, and saith unto him, Eph'-pha-tha, that is, Be opened."

Mark 7:35 "And straightway his ears were opened, and the string of his tongue was loosed, and he spake plain."

*

Mark 8:22 "And he cometh to Beth-sa'-i-da; and they bring a blind man unto him, and besought him to touch him."

Mark 8:23 "And he took the blind man by the hand, and led him out of the town; and when he had spit on his eyes, and put his hands upon him, he asked him if he saw ought."

Mark 8:24 "And he looked up, and said, I see men as trees, walking."

Mark 8:25 "After that he put his hands again upon his eyes, and made him look up: and he was restored, and saw every man clearly."

*

Luke 13:11 "And, behold, there was a woman which had a spirit of infirmity eighteen years, and was bowed together, and could in no wise lift up herself."

Luke 13:12 "And when Jesus saw her, he called her to him, and said unto her, Woman, thou art loosed from thine infirmity.

Luke 13:13 "And he laid his hands on her; and immediately she was made straight, and glorified God."

*

Luke 4.40 "Now when the sun was setting, all they that had any sick with divers diseases brought them unto him; and he laid his hands on every one of them, and healed them."

*

Matthew 20:33 "They say unto him, Lord, that our eyes may be opened."

Matthew 20:34 "So Jesus had compassion on them, and touched their eyes: and immediately their eyes received sight, and they followed him."

*

Luke: 22:51 " And Jesus answered and said, Suffer ye thus far. And he touched his ear, and healed him."

"The Works that I do Shall He (You) do Also"

Jesus declared that the work that he does, you can do also if you believe in him.

John 14.10 '…I speak not of myself: but the father that dwelleth in me, he doeth the works. "

John 14.12 "…I say unto you, He that believeth on me, the works that I do shall he do also: and greater works than these shall he do; because I go unto my father."

John 14.18 "I will not leave you comfortless: I will come to you."

*

Mark 9:23 " ...all things are possible to him that believeth."

Acts in Evidence

The Bible continues to show good deeds that can be done by the Grace of God by others than the Christ. May you this day begin to see how you also can be an instrument of Divine Grace in the lives of many.

Acts 3:6 "Then Peter said, Silver and gold have I none; but such as I have give I thee: In the name of Jesus Christ of Nazareth rise up and walk."

Acts 3:7 "And he took him by the right hand , and lifted him up: and immediately his feet and ancle bones received strength."

Acts 3:8 "And he leaping up stood, and walked, and entered with them into the temple, walking, and leaping, and praising God."

*

Acts 9:17 "And An-a-ni'- as went his way, and entered into the house: and putting his hands on him said, Brother Saul, the Lord, even Jesus, that appeared unto thee in the way as thou camest, hath sent me, that thou mightest receive thy sight, and be filled with the Holy Ghost."

Acts 9:18 And immediately there fell from his eyes as it had been scales: and he received sight forthwith, and arose, and was baptized."

*

Acts 14:8 "And there sat a certain man at Lys'-tra, impotent in his feet, being a cripple from his mother's womb, who never walked:

Acts 14:9 "The same heard Paul speak : who steadfastly beholding him, and perceiving that he had faith to be healed,"

Acts 14:10 "Said with a loud voice, Stand upright on thy feet, And he leaped and walked."

*

Acts 20:9 "And there sat in a widow a certain young man named Eu'-ty-chus, being fallen into a deep sleep: and as Paul was long preaching, he sunk down with sleep, and fell down from the third loft, and was taken up dead."

Acts 20:10 " And Paul went down, and fell on him, and embracing his said, Trouble not yourselves; for his life is in him."

*

And Now,
Will You Accept Your Role in the Divine Plan?
What Can You Do?
What Will You Do?

Chapter Twenty-One

So Where are the Angels?

Humor really helps me when the enemy is trying to divert my focus. You may have noticed that a lot of professional comedians have Jewish roots. Listen and they will tell you their stories.

Growing up in delightfully diverse Philadelphia, I have a lot of experience with many cultures and especially with Jewish folks and black folks. Embracing the joy and pain of friends over the years allows some delicious humor in my head when I am trying to be in spiritual clarity.

Angels and other Beings of the Light can really be an act worthy of television. Picture me being on the Tonight show with Jay leno or Jimmy Fallon and he asks, So where are the Angels in Your Book?

Well the Angels beat him to the question as they appeared this morning in my shower. I thought that I had finished the book yesterday. Right, so here we go again.

I have written down over two hundred messages that have come to me within the last year that have come through a connection that is now called Angel Raphael Speaks. I do not think that any of the messages have been about veterans.

So I answered the question. "You didn't say you wanted to be in the book". And the reply was, "you could have asked. You ask about everything else"

With a shift to a more serious energy, I got a Personal Inner Divine Identity Sign from Angel Ariel. I asked for the meaning, I was told that " There is a problem here in that there is asking, answering, clarity, confusion, trauma, remedy, belief systems and bull stinky stuff.

The power needed by many veterans is merely a self- authority shift which can manifest great rewards. That sounds simple right? Not so fast.

The practitioners that are working with veterans are doing top notch clinical work according to the protocols of their professions. Amplification of the results can be had by spiritual support for existing efforts and the inclusion of optional alternative programs that can have spiritual acceleration.

It is possible Mike for you to start a series of sessions where veterans share their spiritual successes. As they continue to share their healings, they will continue to expand both their healing and their ability to help others realize a connection with the Great Physician who can heal all always."

I should comment that Healing and Curing are quite different and often confused. Healing is a process that can take a while and manifest as something quite different than what is asked for. Curing is the end of an illness process when the goal is attained.

The programs mentioned can be both actual and virtual. Truth that causes resonance with seekers of it can be found both out loud and in print.

"Yo Bro. We axed and you haven't answered the peoples". The answer is coming right up as I follow the directions as quickly as I can.

I should explain about the Angel Raphael Speaks Channelings which started in May of 2013. So far there have been about two hundred messages released free in some twenty-one little e-books which can be found at Internet Joint Ventures.

Most of the messages are also available on my Facebook fan page and at http://www.AngelRaphaelspeaks.com and as e-books at http://www.spiritualcomfortcare.com/angel-raphael-speaks/

So next, I will ask if it is appropriate for me to do a single topic message set for veterans.

Chapter Twenty-Three

A New Single Topic Message Set from the Angel Raphael Speaks Series

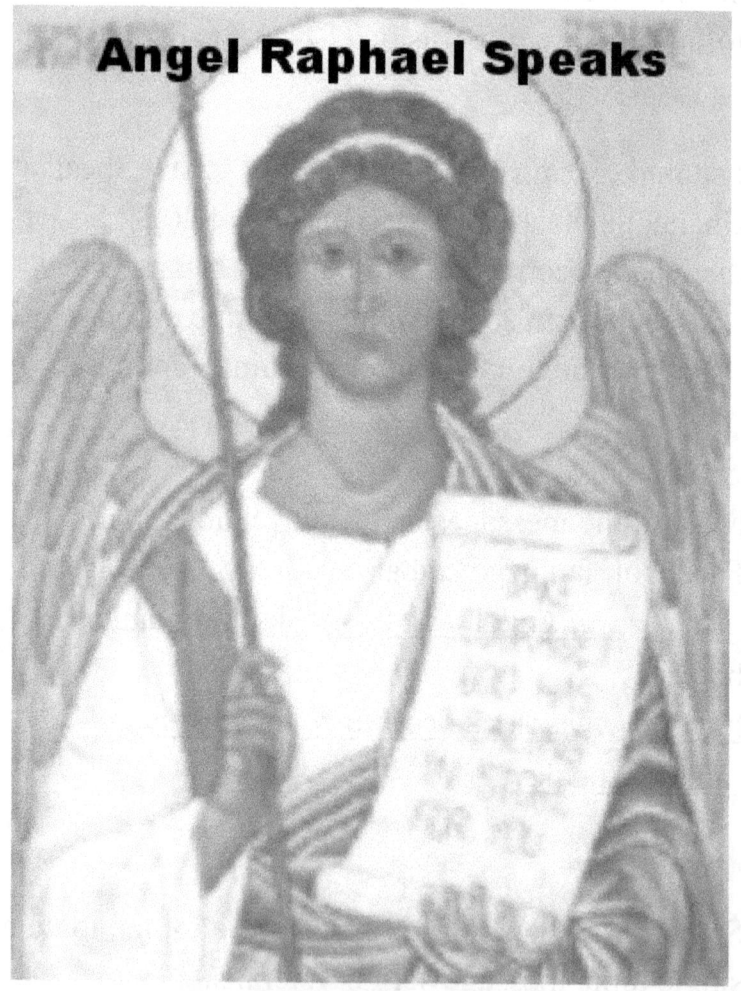

Who is the Veteran Now?

Veterans have served in a role that is not congruent with the truth of their being. They have performed a job as they struggled with the role that they have been assigned.

In the moment of their present existence, they need to be aware that they can choose to move in many directions. This is not to say that they have to choose immediately to be this or that.

Veterans have already experienced many pressures to do many things and as all that has come to a close, there is new freedom available to them.

No Pressure to Act

Being surrounded by loved ones can be wonderful but it can also create new issues for veterans to ponder. Let this be an invitation for each veteran to take the time they need to understand where they are and what they want.

While many questions will be asked of you, allow yourself to not feel pressured to answer. Allow yourself to be drawn to that which brings you peace.

In every moment there is the power of life that can help you to accept where you are and choose what you want. Know that you can take as much time as you need to and then when you are ready, you can move forward with your life.

Disconnection

Many times veterans return to find a world that is different than the way it was or different than the way they thought it was. Do not be alarmed about any changes because you also have changed and the change you see may be better aligned with who you are than you think it is.

The lives of your friends may have continued to change and others may have stepped into relationships or jobs that you once thought were yours. The new reality may be somewhat intimidating at first but closer study will allow you to see that there is still room for you.

As you understand that which is different, know that the new you now has new opportunities to study and grow. The government has many programs to help when you are ready to take advantage of them.

Indecision

It is perfectly normal for veterans to not want to make any decisions. After all, you have been trained to take orders and that became your normal.

Your new normal does not have a personal order giver to tell you how to live your life. While it may feel like you have been abandoned, in reality you have been elevated to a new level of respect that allows you to think independently and be who you want to be and do what you want to do.

While the new found freedom may feel not so great, embracing your freedom can lead to an expansion of your opportunities.

Shame

Strange as it may seem, some veterans can feel a shame for having served in a military situation. Allowing any shame to fall away is hastened when you embrace the support of your creator and the Angels.

When taken into the military, young people have little understanding of the reality of the situation that they are entering. The realities of life can be sobering and survival needs can change many a soul.

If you have an issue that persists, military chaplains and civilian ministers alike are well equipped to help you understand your situation. The situation will not remedy itself so if you are troubled, know that you are worthy of the support you need so be empowered to ask precisely for the help.

Asking is Important

All the Angels and Veteran agencies honor your free will and your independence. Receiving service as a veteran is different than when one is in the military.

Please know emphatically that you are worthy of support in many ways and there is absolutely no reason why you need to hesitate to ask for all that you have earned by being a child of God and a participant in the military forces of your country.

As a Veteran

Knowing what you know brings with it responsibility to share the truth of your convictions. You may be totally at peace with the way your country conducts its' business or you may find that peace is an option that you would like to see pursued.

You can be quiet about your feelings or you may get active in the affairs and organizations of your country so that others can know what you know to be true.

Being a veteran means that you are out of the military but it does not mean that you no longer have any ability to serve your fellow citizens.

As you relax into your life, you will respect fully the value of the journey that you have taken and the importance of all that you have learned. Know the full measure of your significance.

Where Do You Wish to Go Next?

Is there a battle that you have left to fight? Is there a fellow brother or sister from the Military that has had it rougher than you who would be honored to hear from you or be visited by you?

Is there a battle that you feel called to fight which is beckoning you into service of a new kind.

What is there deep within that is calling to your genius and asking you to be all that you can?

Who in your family could use your guidance and support?

Please know that you are still here for a purpose. Finding that purpose can be difficult but when you do, you will find joy that you can share with many more than you can ever imagine.

As Reverend Mike would say, "May all Who Read this be Blessed AND SO IT IS."

Chapter Twenty-Four
Message For Veterans

How to Move Forward

If you still have issues that are holding you back, then it is time for you to get serious about releasing things that no longer serve you. Step one is to try and figure out where you are at present.

A Global Positioning system can easily tell you how to direct your car from where you are to where you want to go. Directing a car is quite direct when you know the origin and destination.

I invite you to experiment with being your own GPS unit for your life. You will need the same things as a GPS Device, your origin and destination.

You establish your origin by writing your present story. Sit down and write the Who, What, When, Where, How and why of where you are now.

Next write the Who, What, When, Where, How and Why of where you want to be at a selected date in the next year. Follow that with further definition for year two and then year three.

Now that you have an origin and destination for your journey, you need to determine how you will get from where you are to where you want to be. You do this by determining what you need in the four parts of your life that I discussed earlier and then claim that support to arrange the life of your dreams.

Depending upon the priority of your issues, your approach can vary widely. Do not be concerned with narrow minded opinions that tend to limit options. Allow yourself to think bigger than you ever have in your life. Use the dreams as fuel to fire your passion.

Determine any preparatory steps that you need to take in the next thirty days before you start. Define your start date and write a plan that you will start to implement then.

Spiritual Healing

I have mentioned earlier that it was spiritual healing that served me well and I invite you to consider using it. Please know there is a subtle and powerful difference between religion and spirituality.

I would encourage you to look locally first to see what is available to you. You may find immediate support that feels good and wholesome and right at the church that you grew up in.

You may also find that the fit is not right for who you are and what you need now. It could be that another nearby church of the same denomination could be the perfect fit for you.

You may need to look around to find the connections that you need. Another source may be other denominations, holistic centers, chiropractic offices, naturopathic doctors and/or health food stores.

Spiritual healing can involve prayer as churches use or it may involve meditation, visualization, bodywork, energy healing, massage, laying on of hands, crystals, stones etc .etc. depending upon the credentials and skills of a practitioner or teacher.

All non-traditional practitioners are not created equal so remember to be careful about going to people who are referred by people that you feel trustworthy.

Reiki

Many who need healing can easily find Reiki in their community and I would encourage you to find out about the Reiki community in your community. It is a great place to start.

If there is a Reiki Share for free or donation/low cost, I would recommend that you check it out and feel how it resonates with you. Do not be alarmed either way, it would be a new experience and your feeling will vary with the individual that you meet. Please do not be quick to judge. Allow yourself to experience, compare and learn anew.

If Reiki speaks to you and you know that it can serve you well, consider taking a course to Reiki Level 1 of the Usui System of Natural Healing which could also be called "Shoden" Level. I suggest the Usui System as it is the most prevalent system in the western world. That makes it easy for you to compare class prices and content expectations.

Emotional Care
Integrated Energy Therapy®

I have already mentioned IET above but I bring it here because, in my view, one of the most critical issues for me and veterans that I have known is the need for the release of stuffed emotions and cellular memory. It matters not whether the stuffed emotions and cellular memory came along with the soul, through life experience or combat intensity, stuffed emotions impede the quality of life and can be worked in many ways to bring options for the peeling of pain, releasing shutdown or reclusiveness.

IET is a trademarked process which helps to keep the treatments aligned with a set protocol. I was privileged to be among the first thirty-four Master Instructors in the world and I am still thrilled with the results of a session that I do for others whether they are right in front of me or across the continent. I have even had marvelous results with doing a session through a translator when the client was on a different continent.

Powerful Information

I know that a lot of veterans do not have resources to see private practitioners so I have created websites that optimize the potential for individuals to learn enough to help themselves.

Please visit my free sites;

http://www.Create-A-Prayer.com

http://www.AngelRaphaelSpeaks.com

http://www.StressReleaseCoach.com

http://www.SpiritualComfortCare.com

http://www.Reiki-Healing.us

http://www.ReverendMikeWanner.com

If I Can Help.

I also offer professional services locally and by distant healing:

Physical and Emotional Healing at
http://LetMeHelpYouHeal.withMike.com

Angel Channeling at
http://www.AngelHealing.withMike.com

Why Are You Still Here?

People ask, Why am I still here? The answer
could vary but likely because your soul's purpose
is not complete and you still have a mission to
complete in this lifetime.

Please know that each of us is loved differently by
the one that created us for our special mission in
this lifetime. You may never know why you were
here or how significant something that you did or
will do is.

The Importance of Now

As you are where you are now, you can choose
how you feel. What you do and don't do are also
choices that you can make. I would suggest that if
you align with the Divine that your time will be
fine.

Have you ever noticed that the creek and rivers have both an upstream and a downstream? That is the perfect metaphor for how we live our lives.

We can go with the flow or we can go against the flow. Many times our lives may have seemed difficult because we may be going against the Divine flow of all that is around us. We can choose to go with the flow at any time in our life.

When we follow the right path for us, all becomes easier than we can imagine and many can benefit from our awareness that encompasses them. We are not here by accident. We are each part of a plan that is beyond our understanding.

What Is A Veteran To Do?

By now, you surely know that I will not insult you by telling you what is right for you because no one has the right to do that but you.

I would like to invite you to own your personal significance and I do not mean that in a bold and boisterous way. I invite you to own the significance of your contribution as it is. Whether you feel it is large or small, I invite you to know that it is what it is.

I also invite your awareness of those that have faired not as well as you and ask if you might be gracious enough to offer any smile you can to everyone that you meet. Some who receive your smile may not have known anywhere near your experience of life. Others that you meet may stop themselves from taking their life because a wise soul like you cared enough to smile on them.

I know not your burden and you know not mine but we all can smile and make the world a better place for all the children of all the nations of a world that we have tried to help by doing the biding of our country previously and the biding of our hearts in every moment since. Blessed be thee now and forever AND SO IT IS by the grace of God Almighty. Thank you noble veteran and carrier of Joy to the World.

ReverendMikeWanner.com

Resource List

Distant Physical Healing from where I am to wherever you are...
http://LetMeHelpYouHeal.withMike.com

Distant Angel Healing from where I am to wherever you are.........
http://AngelHealing.withmike.com/

Services, Products and Websites by Rev. Mike –

Book – Stress Release Energy Work
http://www.Amazon.com
Book - Angel Raphael Speaks Volume One
 http://www.Amazon.com
Book - Angel Raphael Speaks Volume Two
 http://www.Amazon.com
Reiki Journaling From Japan...   http:// www. Amazon.com
Rose Quartz Hearts help the healing focus
http://RoseQuartzHearts.withRevMike.com
Book - Reiki Journaling From Japan
http://www.Amazon.com
Book- Reiki Is Alive   http://www.Amazon.com
Book – Four Parts To Healing   http://www.Amazon.com
Book – Distant Healing   http://www.Amazon.com

Free Resources

Learn to dump fear at
http://TheGreatAmericanFearDump.withMike.com
Spiritually Prepare for Surgery
http://PrepareForSurgery.withRevMike.com
Angel Scribe messages at
http://www.SpiritualComfortCare.com
Law of Attraction Expert column at
http://www.ReverendMikeWanner.com
Stress Release at
http://www.StressReleaseCoach.com

Angel Raphael Speaks through Rev. Mike Wanner. I have channeled multiple message sets and they all have to be polished to smooth out my errors and negotiate some words that may be too easily misunderstood. Grammar is not polished as it is too easy to miss the subtlety of the energy flow. To find out the availability of messages and latest updates go to. http://www.spiritualcomfortcare.com/angel-raphael-speaks/

Also "Tell Mike your concerns – If he and I agree there is a broader need, messages may follow. Citizens of all nations invited as long as your write in English. Do not expect him to answer as he is very busy already listening to us." E-mail Mike at mikewann@voicenet.com.

Rev. Michael Wanner

Rev. Michael Wanner started his metaphysical and ministerial studies with Reiki in 1993 and has studied seven styles of Reiki in the U.S., Japan, Canada, Denmark and Australia. He is certified to teach. He became certified to teach Integrated Energy Therapy in 1999 and co-taught the first IET class of the new Millennium. Mike began dowsing in 2001.

Ordained as a Metaphysical Minister of the International Metaphysical Ministry and an Interfaith Minister of the Circle of Miracles Ministry, Rev. Mike practices and teaches spiritual energy therapies in the Philadelphia Area.

Rev. Mike holds ministerial degrees from the University of Metaphysics and the University of Sedona. He is a Pastoral Care Associate of Aria – Frankford Hospital. He taught at the National Academy of Massage Therapy and Health Sciences.

Rev. Mike was a faculty member of the Medical Mission Sister's Center for Human Integration's School of Integrated Body/Mind Therapies in Fox Chase, Philadelphia, PA for twelve years.

Rev. Mike is licensed by the teaching of Intuitional Metaphysics to practice Spiritual Healing and Scientific Prayer. Mike is also a Prayer therapist.

Rev. Mike was elected in 2007 to the status of "Fellow of the American Institute of Stress."

In 2008, Rev. Mike became a practitioner of Coincidental Recognition as he incorporated the CoRe system in to his spiritual healing practice.

In 2009, Rev. Mike trademarked a new healing process called Quantum Quatro! Subtle Energy System Support®.

In 2011, Rev. Mike joined the outreach program known as the Health Advantage Group.

In 2012. Rev. Mike became a Certified Professional Coach by The Master Coaching Academy and Joined The Personal Empowerment Group .

Prior to his metaphysical, ministerial and coaching studies, Rev. Mike worked for Sears Roebuck and Co. while in High School and after graduation until he joined the U. S. Air Force in 1965. He returned to Sears from Vietnam in 1969 and stayed until 1978. His final Sears assignment was as an efficiency expert in Methods - Operational Research and Development. He volunteered with Burholme Emergency Medical Services from 1969 and is still a Life Member and Board of Directors Member. He started a private ambulance company in 1975 and worked professionally in the field until 2001 when he devoted his full attention to real estate investing, healing and coaching.

*

May All Who Read This Be Blessed
Reverend Mike Wanner
www.ReveredMikeWanner.com
www.AngelRaphaelSpeaks.com
www.StressReleaseCoach.com

www.ingramcontent.com/pod-product-compliance
Lightning Source LLC
Chambersburg PA
CBHW051722170526
45167CB00002B/764